Intermittent Fasting

The Simplest Guide to Master all the secrets of Fasting and Losing weight with intermittent, alternate-day, and extended fasting

Additionally, the information in the following pages is intended only for informational purposes and should thus be thought of as universal. As befitting its nature, it is presented without assurance regarding its prolonged validity or interim quality. Trademarks that are mentioned are done without written consent and can in no way be considered an endorsement from the trademark holder.

Table of Contents

―

BREAKFAST RECIPES

Classic Steak 'n Eggs

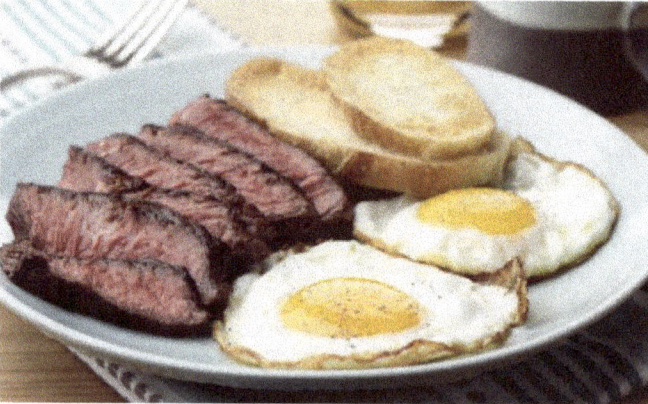

Preparation Time: 5 minutes

Cooking Time: 15 minutes

Servings: 4

Ingredients:

- 8 eggs
- 16-ounces sirloin steak
- 4 tablespoons butter
- ripe avocado
- Salt and pepper to taste

Directions:

1. Melt 2 tbsp. of butter in a huge skillet.
2. Fry eggs 4 at a time until the edges are crispy.
3. While the second batch of eggs are cooking, cook the sirloin in another skillet (with the other 2 tablespoons of butter) until it's at least 160-degrees.
4. Season eggs and steak well with salt and pepper.
5. Serve with slices of avocado.

Nutrition: Total calories: 480 Protein: 37 Carbs: 4 Fat: 37 Fiber: 3

Homemade Sausage, Egg, and Cheese Sandwich

Preparation Time: 5 minutes

Cooking Time: 30 minutes

Servings: 1

Ingredients:

- Muffin
- egg
- 1 tablespoon coconut flour
- 1 tablespoon almond milk
- ½ tablespoon olive oil
- ½-teaspoon baking powder
- Pinch of salt
- Filling
- 1 egg
- ¼-pound breakfast sausage
- 1 slice cheddar cheese

Directions:

1. Preheat oven to 400-degrees.
2. Begin by mixing your muffin batter together first by cracking an egg in a bowl, then mixing in the rest of the ingredients.
3. Grease a ramekin and pour in the batter.
4. Bake for 15 minutes.
5. To get an egg that's the same size as your muffin, crack an egg in a ramekin and whisk.
6. Flavor with salt and pepper, then bake for 10 minutes.

7. For your sausage, just form the meat into a patty.
8. Heat a skillet, and then cook patty for 4-5 minutes per side.
9. When the muffins are ready, remove from oven and carefully slice in half.
10. For a toasty muffin, stick in a toaster for a few minutes.
11. Build sandwich and top with a slice of cheese.
12. Eat!

Nutrition: Total calories: 460 Protein: 29 Carbs: 3 Fat: 37 Fiber: 0

Chicken Sausage Breakfast Casserole

Preparation Time: 10 minutes

Cooking Time: 40 minutes

Servings: 4

Ingredients:

- 1-pound chicken sausage
- 3 big eggs
- 2 cups chopped tomatoes
- 2 cups diced zucchini
- ½ cups cheddar cheese
- ½ cup diced onion
- ½ cup plain Greek yogurt
- 1 teaspoon dried sage
- 1 teaspoon dried mustard

Directions:

1. Preheat oven to 375-degrees.
2. Preheat a skillet until warm, then add sausage.
3. When nearly all the pink is gone, put the zucchini and onion.
4. Cook until the veggies are softened.
5. Move skillet contents to a greased casserole dish.
6. In a separate bowl, mix eggs, yogurt, and seasonings together.
7. Lastly, mix one cup of cheese into eggs.
8. Pour into the casserole dish on top of the sausage and veggies.

9. Bake for at least 30 minutes until cheese has melted and starts browning.
10. Serve right away!

Nutrition: Total calories: 487 Protein: 19 Carbs: 4.8 Fat: 42 Fiber: 1.3

Cheddar-Chive Omelet for One

Preparation Time:8 minutes

Cooking Time: 5 minutes

Servings: 1

Ingredients:

- 2 slices cooked bacon
- 2 big eggs
- 2 stalks chives
- 2 tablespoons sharp cheddar cheese
- teaspoon olive oil
- Salt and pepper to taste

Directions:

1. Heat oil in a skillet.
2. While that heats, chop chives.
3. Pour in eggs and sprinkle chives, salt, and pepper on top.
4. Wait until edges are beginning to set.
5. Crumble bacon on top and wait another 25 seconds.
6. Remove skillet from heat.
7. Sprinkle on cheese and carefully fold omelet over.
8. Enjoy!

Nutrition: Total calories: 463 Protein: 24 Carbs: 1 Fat: 39 Fiber: 1

Breakfast-Stuffed Bell Peppers

Preparation Time: 25 minutes

Cooking Time: 10 minutes

Servings: 4

Ingredients:

- 4 large yellow bell peppers
- 4 eggs
- 4 bacon strips
- 4-ounces pork breakfast sausage
- cup shredded mozzarella cheese
- ½ cup diced onion
- 1 tablespoon minced garlic
- Couple teaspoons olive oil
- Salt and pepper to taste

Directions:

1. Preheat your oven to 275-degrees.
2. Chop the tops off the peppers and hollow out the insides.
3. Set on a baking sheet and brush insides with a little olive oil.
4. Stick peppers in the oven.
5. Heat a skillet and cook bacon and sausage until nearly done.
6. Add onions and garlic.
7. Cook until onions have softened.
8. Take out the peppers and stuff.
9. Top with cheese and press down with a spoon, creating a little hollow.

10. Crack in an egg.
11. Turn oven up to 325-degrees and put stuffed peppers in the oven for 10 minutes, or until eggs have reached the doneness you like.
12. Serve!

Nutrition: Total calories: 372 Protein: 27 Carbs: 15 Fat: 24 Fiber: 2

Avocado Stuffed with Tuna

Preparation Time: 20 minutes

Cooking Time: 0 minutes

Servings: 2

Ingredients:

- avocado
- 1 can of tuna
- 1 tomato
- ½ onion
- Parsley to taste

Directions:

1. Cut the avocado into halves. Remove the middle parts so that you can have a room for stuffing. (Keep the "meat" parts)
2. Cut the tomato and onion into tiny circles.
3. Mix meat parts with tuna, tomato, and onion.
4. Stuff the avocado halves with the mixture, decorate with parsley to taste and serve!

Nutrition: Calories: 132 Fats: 3g Net Carbs: 6g Protein: 1.2g Fiber: 7g

Tuna in Cucumber

Preparation Time: 15 minutes

Cooking Time: 0 minutes

Servings: 6

Ingredients:

- cucumber
- ½ celery leaf
- ½ red bell pepper
- 1 can of tuna
- Pepper and salt to taste

Directions:

1. Peel the cucumber and cut it into thicker circles. Make a hole in each piece.
2. Cut the celery and pepper into tiny cubes. Mix them with tuna.
3. Put 1 tbsp. of tuna mixture into cucumbers.
4. Add spices to taste and serve.
5. Enjoy!

Nutrition: Calories: 109 Total Fats: 1.6g Net Carbs: 4g Protein: 1g Fiber: 5.4g

Small Intermittent Pies

Preparation Time: 10 minutes

Cooking Time: 30 minutes

Servings: 6

Ingredients:

- 3 eggs
- 5 bacon slices
- ½ red bell pepper
- leek
- ½ cup of broccoli
- oz. of ground cheese
- ½ cup of yogurt
- ¼ pack of baking powder
- tbsp. of olive oil
- Salt, pepper, powdered garlic, parsley to taste

Directions:

1. Whisk and blend the eggs with baking powder.
2. Cook the broccoli in water.
3. Cut bacon, leek and pepper into smaller pieces to taste.
4. Mix cheese with yogurt well. Then, add bacon, leek, pepper, and spices to taste.
5. Join the 2 mixtures together and then pour into cupcake or muffin molds.
6. Bake for 30 minutes at 200°F.

Nutrition: Calories: 121 Total Fats: 2.1g Net Carbs: 2g Protein: 1.3g Fiber: 6g

LUNCH RECIPES

Kabobs with Peanut Curry Sauce

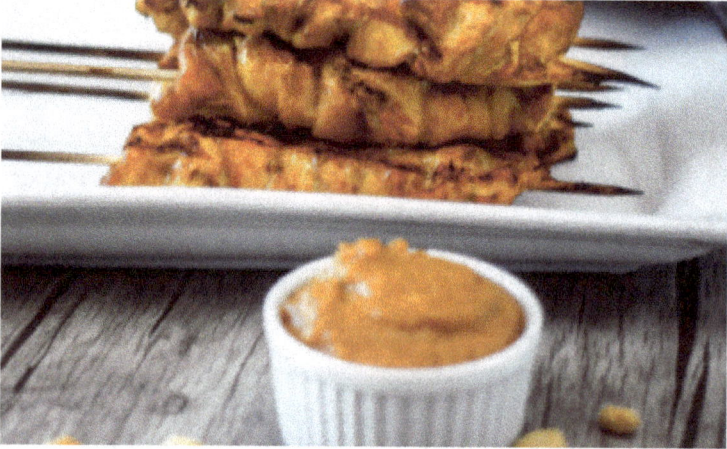

Preparation Time: 9 minutes

Cooking Time: 9 minutes

Servings: 4

Ingredients:

- 1 cup Cream
- 4 tsp Curry Powder
- 1 1/2 tsp Cumin
- 1 1/2 tsp Salt
- 1 T minced garlic
- 1/3 cup Peanut Butter, sugar-free
- 2 T Lime Juice
- 3 T Water
- 1/2 small Onion, diced
- 2 T Soy Sauce
- 1 packet Splenda
- 8 oz. boneless, cooked Chicken Breast
- 8 oz. pork tenderloin

Directions:

1. Blend together cream, onion, 2 tsp. garlic, curry and cumin powder, and salt.

2. Slice the meats into 1-inch pieces.

3. Place the cream sauce into a bowl and put in the chicken and tenderloin to marinate. Let rest in sauce for 14 minutes.

4. Blend peanut butter, water, 1 tsp. garlic, lime juice, soy sauce, and Splenda. This is your peanut dipping sauce.

5. Remove the meats and thread on skewers. Broil or grill 4 minutes per side until meat is done.

6. Serve with dipping sauce.

Nutrition: Calories: 530 Total Fat: 29g Protein: 37g Total Carbs: 6g Dietary Fiber: 4g Sugar: 2g Sodium: 1538mg

Pizza

Preparation Time: 4 minutes

Cooking Time: 4 minutes

Servings: 1

Ingredients:

- 1 Tortilla Factory low carb whole wheat tortilla

- ¼ cup mozzarella cheese, hand-shredded

- ¼ cup tomato paste

- sprinkle of Italian seasoning

- sprinkle of garlic salt

- Cut the broccoli, spinach, mushrooms, peppers, and onions you like for toppings

Directions:

1. Turn broiler on in oven, or toaster oven

2. Spread tortilla with tomato paste

3. Sprinkle seasoning on the paste

4. Add the cheese

5. Add the veggies

6. Broil or toast 1-4 minutes until crust is crunchy and cheese melted

Nutrition: Calories: 155 Total Fat: 7g Protein: 13g Total Carbs: 18g Dietary Fiber: 10g Sugar: 2g Sodium: 741mg

Salmon with Bok-Choy

Preparation Time: 9 minutes

Cooking Time: 9 minutes

Servings: 4

Ingredients:

- 1 c red peppers, roasted, drained
- 2 cups chopped bok-choy
- 1 T salted butter
- 5 oz. salmon steak
- 1 lemon, sliced very thinly
- 1/8 tsp black pepper
- 1 T olive oil
- 2 T sriracha sauce

Directions:

1. Place oil in skillet
2. Place all but 4 slices of lemon in the skillet.
3. Sprinkle the bok choy with the black pepper.
4. Stir fry the bok-choy with the lemons.
5. Remove and place on four plates.

6. Place the butter in the skillet and stir fry the salmon, turning once.

7. Place the salmon on the bed of bok-choy.

8. Divide the red peppers and encircle the salmon.

9. Place a slice of lemon atop the salmon.

10. Drizzle with sriracha sauce.

Nutrition: Calories: 410 Total Fat: 30g Protein: 30g Total Carbs: 7g Dietary Fiber: 2g Sugar: 0g Sodium: 200mg

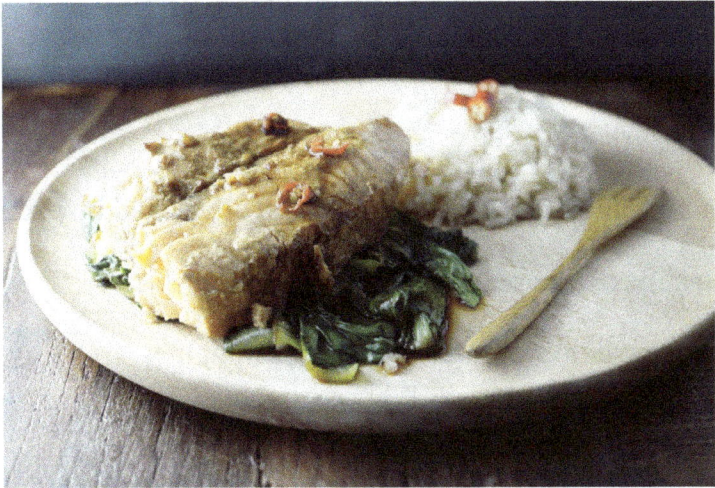

31

Sriracha Tuna Kabobs

Preparation Time: 4 minutes

Cooking Time: 9 minutes

Servings: 4

Ingredients:

- 4 T Huy Fong chili garlic sauce
- 1 T sesame oil infused with garlic
- 1 T ginger, fresh, grated
- 1 T garlic, minced
- 1 red onion, cut into quarters and separated by petals
- 2 cups bell peppers, red, green, yellow
- 1 can whole water chestnuts, cut in half
- ½ pound fresh mushrooms, halved
- 32 oz. boneless tuna, chunks or steaks
- 1 Splenda packet
- 2 zucchini, sliced 1 inch thick, keep skins on

Directions:

1. Layer the tuna and the vegetable pieces evenly onto 8 skewers.

2. Combine the spices and the oil and chili sauce, add the Splenda

3. Quickly blend, either in blender or by quickly whipping.

4. Brush onto the kabob pieces, make sure every piece is coated

5. Grill 4 minutes on each side, check to ensure the tuna is cooked to taste.

6. Serving size is two skewers.

Nutrition: Calories: 467 Total Fat: 18g Protein: 56g Total Carbs: 21g Dietary Fiber: 3.5g Sugar: 6g Sodium: 433mg

Steak Salad with Asian Spice

Preparation Time: 4 minutes

Cooking Time: 4 minutes

Servings: 2

Ingredients:

- 2 T sriracha sauce

- 1 T garlic, minced

- 1 T ginger, fresh, grated

- 1 bell pepper, yellow, cut in thin strips

- 1 bell pepper, red, cut in thin strips

- 1 T sesame oil, garlic

- 1 Splenda packet

- ½ tsp curry powder

- ½ tsp rice wine vinegar

- 8 oz. of beef sirloin, cut into strips

- 2 cups baby spinach, stemmed

- ½ head butter lettuce, torn or chopped into bite-sized pieces

Directions:

1. Place the garlic, sriracha sauce, 1 tsp sesame oil, rice wine vinegar, and Splenda into a bowl and combine well.

2. Pour half of this mix into a zip-lock bag. Add the steak to marinade while you are preparing the salad.

3. Assemble the brightly colored salad by layering in two bowls.

4. Place the baby spinach into the bottom of the bowl.

5. Place the butter lettuce next.

6. Mix the two peppers and place on top.

7. Remove the steak from the marinade and discard the liquid and bag.

8. Heat the sesame oil and quickly stir fry the steak until desired doneness, it should take about 3 minutes.

9. Place the steak on top of the salad.

10. Drizzle with the remaining dressing (other half of marinade mix).

11. Sprinkle sriracha sauce across the salad.

Nutrition: Calories: 350 Total Fat: 23g Protein: 28g Total Carbs: 7g Dietary Fiber: 3.5 Sugar: 0 Sodium: 267mg

Tilapia and Broccoli

Preparation Time: 4 minutes

Cooking Time: 14 minutes

Servings: 1

Ingredients:

- 6 oz. tilapia, frozen is fine

- 1 T butter

- 1 T garlic, minced or finely chopped

- 1 tsp of lemon pepper seasoning

- 1 cup broccoli florets, fresh or frozen, but fresh will be crisper

Directions:

1. Set the pre-warmed oven for 350 degrees.

2. Place the fish in an aluminum foil packet.

3. Arrange the broccoli around the fish to make an attractive arrangement.

4. Sprinkle the lemon pepper on the fish.

5. Close the packet and seal, bake for 14 minutes.

6. Combine the garlic and butter. Set aside.

7. Remove the packet from the oven and transfer ingredients to a plate.

8. Place the butter on the fish and broccoli.

Nutrition: Calories: 362 Total Fat: 25g Protein: 29g Total Carbs: 3.5g Dietary Fiber: 3g Sugar: 0g Sodium: 0mg

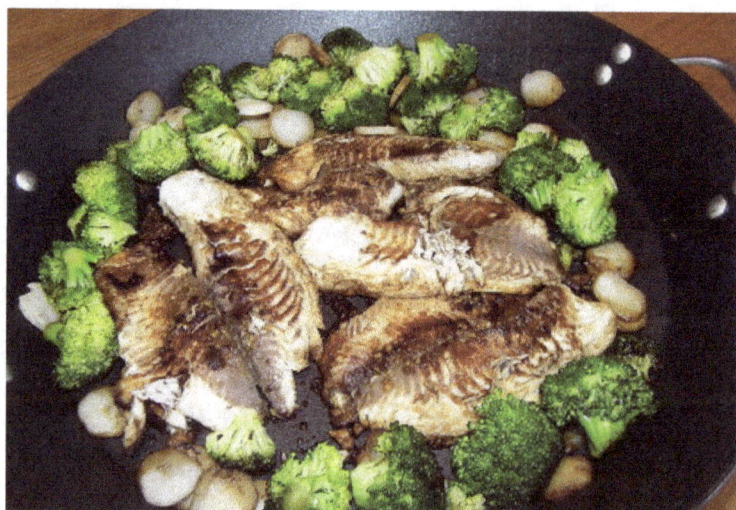

Turkey Salad

Preparation Time: 5 minutes

Cooking Time: 0 minutes

Servings: 4

Ingredients:

- 1 cup cherry tomatoes, halved

- 1 cucumber, sliced

- 1 carrot, grated

- Salt and black pepper to the taste

- 1 tablespoon balsamic vinegar

- 1 tablespoon olive oil

- 1 and ½ cups turkey breast, cooked, skinless, boneless and shredded

Directions:

1. In a salad bowl, combine the turkey with the tomatoes, cucumber and the other ingredients, toss and serve for lunch.

Nutrition: Calories 57 Fat 3.7 Fiber 1.3 Carbs 6.1 Protein 1.2

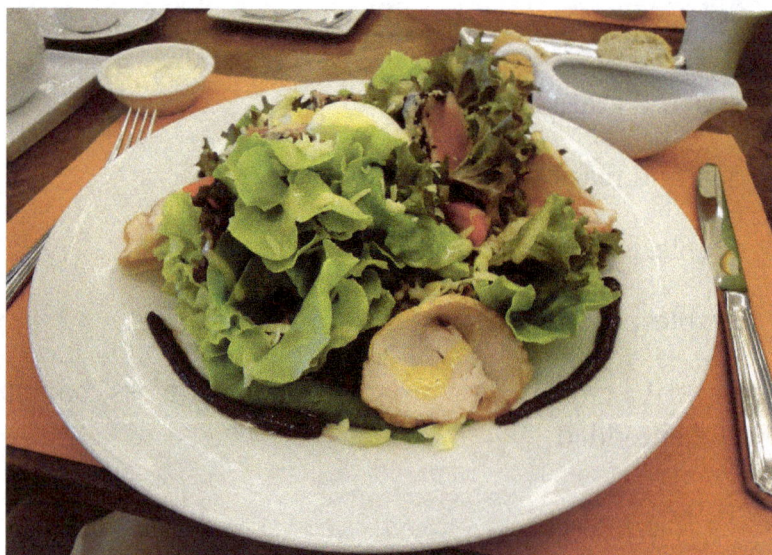

Cheesy Turkey Pan

Preparation Time: 10 minutes

Cooking Time: 25 minutes

Servings: 4

Ingredients:

- 2 cups cheddar cheese, grated
- 1 big turkey breast, skinless, boneless and cubed
- 1 tablespoon tomato passata
- ¼ cup veggie stock
- 1 tablespoon olive oil
- 2 shallots, chopped
- ¼ cup tomatoes, cubed
- Salt and black pepper to the taste

Directions:

1. Ensure that you heat the pan; add the shallots and sauté for 2 minutes.
2. Add the meat and brown for 5 minutes.
3. Add the pasta and the other ingredients except the cheese toss then cook over medium heat for 10 minutes more.
4. Sprinkle the cheese on top, cook everything for 7-8 minutes, divide between plates and serve for lunch.

Nutrition: Calories 309 Fat 23.1 Fiber 0.4 Carbs 3.9 Protein 21.6

Chicken and Leeks Pan

Preparation Time: 10 minutes

Cooking Time: 20 minutes

Servings: 4

Ingredients:

- 2 tablespoons olive oil
- 1-pound chicken breast, skinless, boneless and cut into strips
- 2 shallots, chopped
- 1 cup mozzarella cheese, shredded
- 2 leeks, sliced
- ½ cup veggie stock
- 1 tablespoon heavy cream
- 1 teaspoon sweet paprika
- Salt and black pepper to the taste

Directions:

1. Ensure that you heat the pan, add the shallots, stir then cook for 3 minutes.

2. Add the meat and the leeks, stir and brown for 7 minutes more.

3. Add the other ingredients except the cheese and stir.

4. Sprinkle the cheese on top, introduce the pan in the oven then cook everything at 400 degrees F for 10 minutes more.

5. Divide the mix between plates and serve.

Nutrition: Calories 253 Fat 12.9 Fiber 1 Carbs 7.2 Protein 26.9

Chicken and Peppers Mix

Preparation Time: 10 minutes

Cooking Time: 25 minutes

Servings: 4

Ingredients:

- 1 cup red bell peppers, cut into strips
- 1-pound chicken breast, skinless, boneless and roughly cubed
- 2 spring onions, chopped
- 2 tablespoons olive oil
- 1 tomato, cubed
- Salt and black pepper to the taste
- ¼ cup tomato passata
- 1 tablespoon cilantro, chopped

Directions:

1. Ensure that you heat the pan, add the spring onions and sauté them for 2 minutes.

2. Add the chicken and the bell peppers, stir then cook everything for 8 minutes more.

3. Add the rest of the ingredients, bring to a simmer then cook over medium heat for 15 minutes more stirring often.

4. Divide the mix between plates and serve

Nutrition: Calories 206 Fat 10 Fiber 0.9 Carbs 3.7 Protein 24.8

SIDE DIESHES

Tasty Cauliflower and Mint Rice

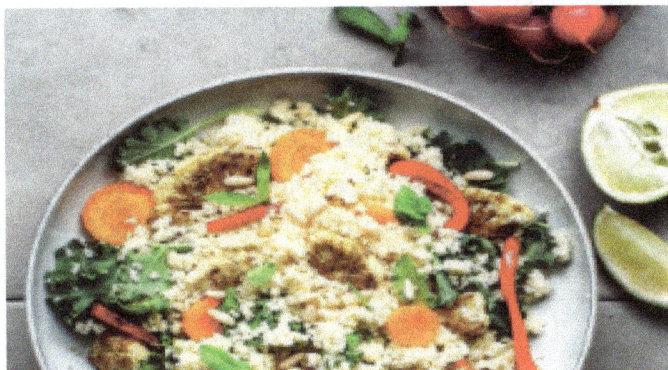

Preparation time: 10 minutes

Cooking time: 5 minutes

Servings: 4

Ingredients:

- cup cauliflower rice
- tablespoons olive oil
- small yellow onion, chopped
- and ½ cups veggie stock
- tablespoons mint, chopped
- A pinch of salt and black pepper

Directions:

1. Set your instant pot on sauté mode, add the oil, heat it up, add onion, stir and cook for 3 minutes.
2. Add veggie stock, cauliflower rice, salt and pepper, stir, cover and cook on High for 5 minutes.
3. Add mint, toss everything to coat, divide between plates and serve right away as a side dish.
4. Enjoy!

Nutrition: Calories 160, fat 3, fiber 2, carbs 6, protein 10

MEATS RECIPES

Sausage and Marinara Casserole

Preparation time: 5 minutes

Cooking time: 12 minutes

Servings: 2

Ingredients:

- 2 oz chorizo
- 4 oz sausage
- tbsp avocado oil
- 4 oz marinara sauce
- tbsp grated cheddar cheese
- ¼ tsp salt
- 1/8 tsp ground black pepper
- ¼ tsp dried thyme

Directions:

1. Take a medium skillet pan, place it over medium heat, add oil and when hot, add chorizo and sausage and cook for 4 to 5 minutes until meat is no longer pink.
2. Add the marinara sauce into the pan, stir in salt, black pepper, and thyme, cook for 1 minute until hot and then transfer meat mixture into a casserole dish.
3. Sprinkle cheese over the top of casserole and then bake for 7 minutes until thoroughly cooked.
4. Serve.

Nutrition: 485 Calories; 44.4 g Fats; 15.6 g Protein; 3.7 g Net Carb; 1.1 g Fiber;

Double Cheese Meatloaf

Preparation time: 10 minutes

Cooking time: 20 minutes

Servings: 2

Ingredients:

- 2 slices of bacon, chopped, cooked
- 6 oz of sausage
- 2 tbsp grated mozzarella cheese
- 2 tbsp grated cheddar cheese
- 1/3 tsp salt
- 1/4 tsp ground black pepper
- tsp dried parsley
- tbsp marinara sauce
- egg

Directions:

1. Turn on the oven, then set it to 375 degrees F and let it preheat.
2. Meanwhile, take a medium bowl, place all the ingredients in it except for marinara and stir until well combined.
3. Spoon the mixture into a mini loaf pan, top with marinara, and then bake for 20 to 25 minutes until cooked through and done.
4. When done, let meatloaf cool for 5 minutes, then cut it into slices and then serve.

Nutrition: 578 Calories; 50.6 g Fats; 27.4 g Protein; 2.6 g Net Carb; 0.3 g Fiber;

Spinach Sausage Ball Pasta

Preparation time: 10 minutes

Cooking time: 12 minutes

Servings: 2

Ingredients:

- pound cabbage, shredded
- 4 oz sausage
- oz spinach, chopped
- tbsp grated parmesan cheese
- 2 tbsp marinara sauce
- 1/3 tsp salt
- ¼ tsp ground black pepper
- 2 tbsp avocado oil

Directions:

1. Take a medium bowl, place sausage in it, add spinach and cheese in it, season with 1/3 tsp salt and black pepper, stir until well combined, and then shape the mixture into balls.
2. Take a medium skillet pan, place it over medium heat, add 1 tbsp oil and when hot, add meatballs and cook for 3 to 4 minutes per side until cooked and nicely golden brown.
3. When transfer meatballs to a plate, add remaining oil into the pan and, when hot, add cabbage and then cook for 3 minutes until tender-crisp.
4. Return meatballs into the pan, add marinara sauce, toss until well mixed and cook for 1 minute until hot. Serve.

Nutrition: 505 Calories; 41.6 g Fats; 18.7 g Protein; 6.5 g Net Carb; 6 g Fiber;

POULTRY

Chicken and Peanut Stir-Fry

Preparation time: 5 minutes

Cooking time: 0

Servings: 2

Ingredients:

- 2 chicken thighs, cubed
- ½ cup broccoli florets
- ¼ cup peanuts
- tbsp sesame oil
- ½ tbsp soy sauce
- Seasoning:
- ½ tsp garlic powder

Directions:

1. Take a skillet pan, place it over medium heat, add ½ tbsp oil and when hot, add chicken cubes and cook for 4 minutes until browned on all sides.
2. Then add broccoli florets and continue cooking for 2 minutes until tender-crisp.
3. Add remaining ingredients, stir well and cook for another 2 minutes.
4. Serve.

Nutrition: 266 Calories; 19 g Fats; 18.5 g Protein; 4 g Net Carb; 2.5 g Fiber;

Chicken Scarpariello with Spicy Sausage

Preparation Time: 10 minutes

Cooking Time: 45 minutes

Servings: 6

Ingredients:

- pound boneless chicken thighs
- Sea salt, for seasoning
- Freshly ground black pepper, for seasoning
- tablespoons good-quality olive oil, divided
- ½ pound Italian sausage (sweet or hot)
- tablespoon minced garlic
- pimiento, chopped
- ¼ cup dry white wine
- cup chicken stock
- tablespoons chopped fresh parsley

Directions:

1. Preheat the oven. Set the oven temperature to 425°F.
2. Brown the chicken and sausage. Pat the chicken thighs to dry using paper towels and season them lightly with salt and pepper. In a large oven-safe skillet over medium-high heat, warm 2 tablespoons of the olive oil. Add the chicken thighs and sausage to the skillet and brown them on all sides, turning them carefully, about 10 minutes.
3. Bake the chicken and sausage. Bring the skillet into the oven and bake for 25 minutes or until the chicken is cooked through. Take the skillet out of the oven, transfer

the chicken and sausage to a plate, and put the skillet over medium heat on the stovetop.

4. Make the sauce. Warm the remaining 1 tablespoon of olive oil, add the garlic and pimiento and sauté for 3 minutes. Pour the white wine and deglaze the skillet by using a spoon to scrape up any browned bits from the bottom of the skillet. Pour in the chicken stock and bring it to a boil, then reduce the heat to low and simmer until the sauce reduces by about half, about 6 minutes.

5. Finish and serve. Put back the chicken and sausage to the skillet, toss it to coat it with the sauce, and serve it topped with the parsley.

Nutrition: Calories: 370 Total fat: 30g Total carbs: 3g Fiber: 0g Net carbs: 3g Sodium: 314mg Protein: 19g

Almond Chicken Cutlets

Preparation Time: 10 minutes

Cooking Time: 15 minutes

Servings: 4

Ingredients:

- 2 eggs
- ½ teaspoon garlic powder
- cup almond flour
- tablespoon chopped fresh oregano
- 4 (4-ounce) boneless skinless chicken breasts, pounded to about ¼ inch thick
- ¼ cup good-quality olive oil
- tablespoons grass-fed butter

Directions:

1. Bread the chicken. Whisk together the eggs, garlic powder in a medium bowl, and set it aside. Stir together the almond flour and oregano on a plate and set the plate next to the egg mixture. Pat the chicken breasts to dry using paper towels and dip them into the egg mixture. Remove excess egg then roll the chicken in the almond flour until they are coated.
2. Fry the chicken. In a large skillet over medium-high heat, warm the olive oil and butter. Add the breaded chicken breasts and fry them, turning them once, until they are cooked through, very crispy, and golden brown, and 14 to 16 minutes in total.

3. Serve. Place one cutlet on each of four plates and serve them immediately.

Nutrition: Calories: 328 Total fat: 23g Total carbs: 0g Fiber: 0g Net carbs: 0g Sodium: 75mg Protein: 28g

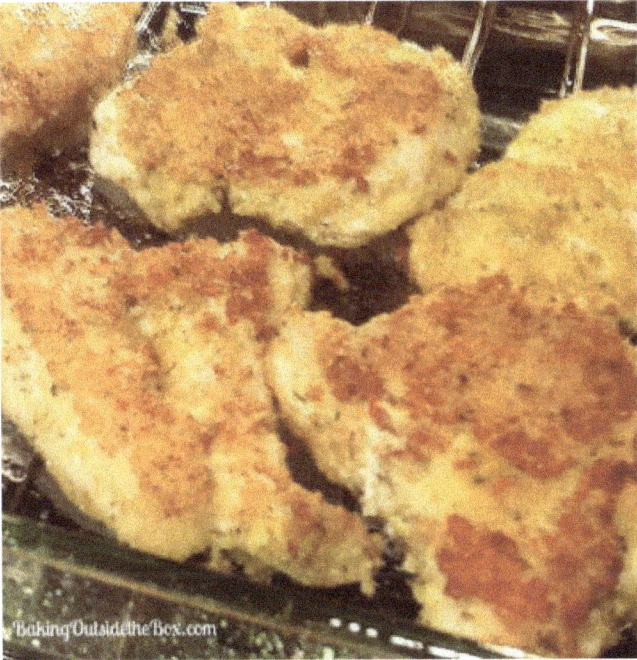

BakingOutsideTheBox.com

Slow Cooker Chicken Cacciatore

Preparation Time: 15 minutes

Cooking Time: 10 minutes

Servings: 4

Ingredients:

- ¼ cup good-quality olive oil
- 4 (4-ounce) boneless chicken breasts, each cut into three pieces
- onion, chopped
- celery stalks, chopped
- cup sliced mushrooms
- tablespoons minced garlic
- (28-ounce) can sodium-free diced tomatoes
- ½ cup red wine
- ½ cup tomato paste
- tablespoon dried basil
- teaspoon dried oregano
- ⅛ teaspoon red pepper flakes

Directions:

1. Brown the chicken. In a skillet at medium-high heat, warm the olive oil. Add the chicken breasts and brown them, turning them once, about 10 minutes in total.
2. Cook in the slow cooker. Place the chicken in the slow cooker and stir in the onion, celery, mushrooms, garlic, tomatoes, red wine, tomato paste, basil, oregano, and red pepper flakes. Cook it on high for approximately 3 to 4

hours or on low for 6 to 8 hours, until the chicken is fully cooked and tender.

3. Serve. Divide the chicken and sauce between four bowls and serve it immediately.

Nutrition: Calories: 383 Total fat: 26g Total carbs: 11g Fiber: 4g Net carbs: 7g Sodium: 116mg Protein: 26g

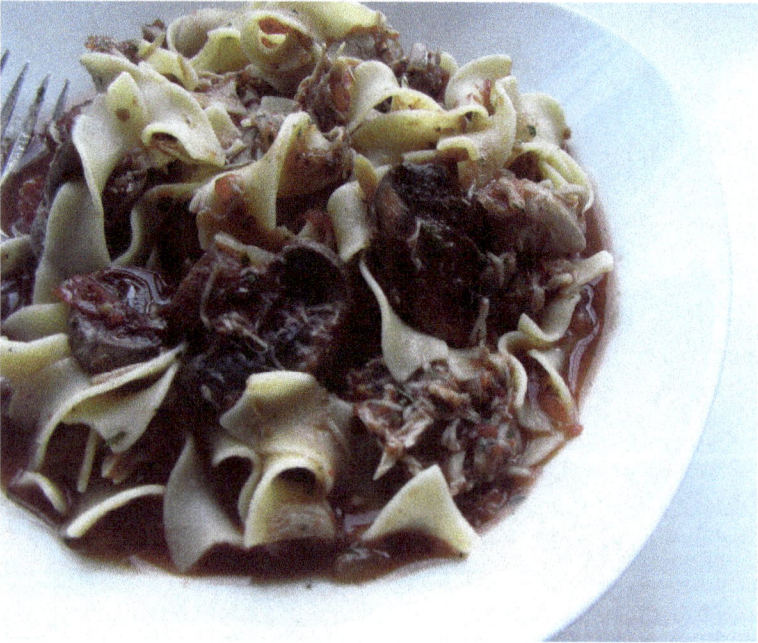

SEAFOOD RECIPES

Glazed Halibut Steak

Preparation Time: 10 minutes

Cooking Time: 15 minutes

Servings: 3

Ingredients:

- lb. halibut steak
- 2/3 cup low-sodium soy sauce
- ½ cup mirin
- tbsp. lime juice
- ¼ cup stevia
- ¼ tsp. crushed red pepper flakes
- ¼ cup orange juice
- garlic clove, smashed
- ¼ tsp. ginger, ground

Directions:

1. Make the teriyaki glaze by mixing all of the ingredients except for the halibut in a saucepan.
2. Place it to a boil and lower the heat, continually stirring until the mixture reduces by half. Take off from the heat and leave to cool.
3. Pour half of the cooled glaze into a Ziploc bag. Add in the halibut, making sure to coat it well in the sauce. Place in the refrigerator for 30 minutes.

———

4. Preheat the Air Fryer to 390°F.
5. Put the marinated halibut in the fryer and allow it to cook for 10 – 12 minutes.
6. Use any the remaining glaze to brush the halibut steak with lightly.
7. Serve with white rice or shredded vegetables.

Nutrition: Calories: 357 kcal Protein: 29.34 g Fat: 23.16 g Carbohydrates: 7.15 g

Tilapia Fillets

Preparation Time: 10 minutes

Cooking Time: 15 minutes

Servings: 3

Ingredients:

- lb. tilapia fillets, sliced
- 4 wheat buns
- egg yolks
- tbsp. fish sauce
- tbsp. mayonnaise
- sweet pickle relish
- tbsp. hot sauce
- tbsp. nectar

Directions:

1. In a bowl, put and whisk the egg yolks and fish sauce.
2. Throw in the mayonnaise, sweet pickle relish, hot sauce, and nectar.
3. Transfer the mixture to a round baking tray.
4. Put it in the Air Fryer and line the sides with the tilapia fillets. Cook for 15 minutes at 300°F.
5. Remove and serve on hamburger buns if desired.

Nutrition: Calories: 248 kcal Protein: 35.29 g Fat: 10.79 g Carbohydrates: 2.15 g

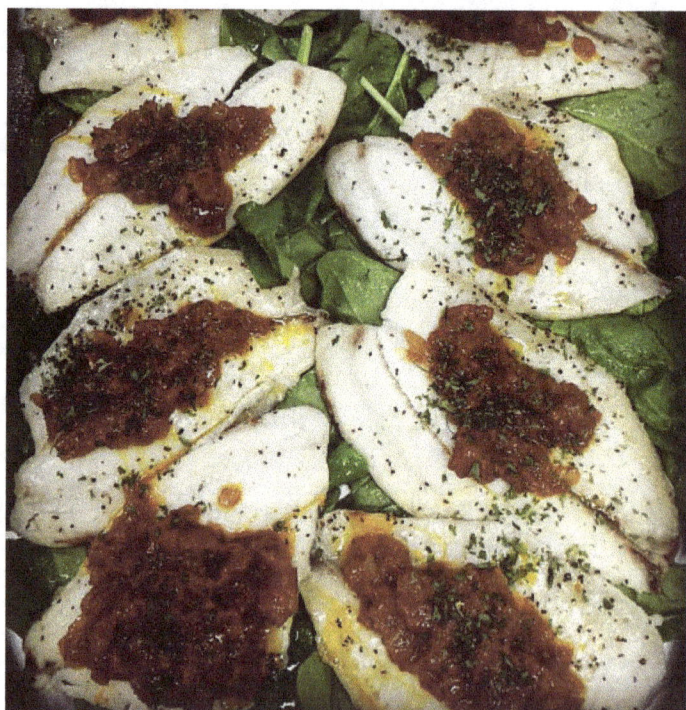

Fish Fingers

Preparation Time: 10 minutes

Cooking Time: 40 minutes

Servings: 2

Ingredients:

- 2 eggs
- 10 oz. Fish, such as mackerel, cut into fingers
- ½ tsp. Turmeric Powder
- ½ Lemon, juiced
- + 1 tsp. mixed dried herbs
- + 1 tsp. Garlic Powder, separately
- ½ tsp. Red Chili Flakes
- cup intermittent-friendly bread crumbs
- tbsp. Maida
- tsp. Intermittent almond flour
- ¼ tsp. baking soda
- tsp. Ginger garlic paste
- ½ tsp. Black pepper
- ½ tsp. sea salt
- – 2 tbsp. olive oil
- Ketchup or tartar sauce [optional]

Directions:

1. Put the fish fingers in a bowl. Cover with 1 teaspoon of mixed herbs, 1 teaspoon of garlic powder, salt, red chili flakes, turmeric powder, black pepper, ginger garlic paste, and lemon juice. Leave to absorb for approximately 10 minutes.

2. In a separate bowl, mix the intermittent almond flour and baking soda. Beat the eggs in the mixture and stir again.
3. Throw in the marinated fish and set aside again for at least 10 minutes.
4. Combine the bread crumbs and the remaining teaspoon of mixed herbs and teaspoon of garlic powder.
5. Roll the fish sticks with the bread crumb and herb mixture.
6. Preheat the Air Fryer at 360°F.
7. Line the basket of the fryer with a sheet of aluminum foil. Place the fish fingers inside the fryer and pour over a drizzle of the olive oil.
8. Cook for 10 minutes, ensuring the fish is brown and crispy before serving. Enjoy with ketchup or tartar sauce if desired.

Nutrition: Calories: 534 kcal Protein: 40.85 g Fat: 34.52 g Carbohydrates: 13.52 g

Intermittent Salmon Tandoori with cucumber sauce

Preparation Time: 15 minutes

Cooking Time: 20 minutes

Servings: 4

Ingredients:

- 25 ounces salmon (bite-sized pieces)
- 2 tablespoons coconut oil
- tablespoon tandoori seasoning
- For the cucumber sauce
- 1/2 shredded cucumber (squeeze out the water completely)
- Juice of 1/2 lime
- minced garlic cloves
- 1/4 cup sour cream or mayonnaise
- 1/2 teaspoon salt (optional)
- For the crispy salad
- 1/2 ounces lettuce (torn)
- scallions (finely chopped)
- avocados (cubed)
- yellow bell pepper (diced)
- Juice of 1 lime

Directions:

1. Preheat the oven to 350 degrees Fahrenheit
2. Mix the tandoori seasoning with oil in a small bowl and coat the salmon pieces with this mixture.

3. Line the baking tray using parchment paper and spread the coated salmon pieces in it.
4. Bake for 20 minutes until soft and the salmon flakes with a fork
5. Take another bowl and place the shredded cucumber in it. Add the mayonnaise, minced garlic, and salt (if the mayonnaise doesn't have salt) to the shredded cucumber. Mix well. Squeeze the lime juice at the top and set the cucumber sauce aside.
6. Mix the lettuce, scallions, avocados, and bell pepper in another bowl. Drizzle the contents with the lime juice.
7. Transfer the veggie salad to a plate and place the baked salmon over it. Top the veggies and salmon with cucumber sauce.
8. Serve immediately and enjoy!

Nutrition: Calories 847 Kcal Fat: 73 g Protein: 35 g Net carb: 6 g

Crab Stuffed Salmon

Preparation Time: 10 minutes

Cooking Time: 30 minutes

Servings: 8

Ingredients:

- 2 lbs. Salmon (wider filet works best)
- 2 tsp Lemon zest
- 2 tbsp. Butter (melted)
- Sea salt
- Black pepper
- Crab Filling:
- 8 oz. Lump crab meat
- 1/2 large onion (chopped)
- 2 tbsp. Mayonnaise
- 2 tbsp. Fresh parsley (chopped)
- 2 cloves Garlic (minced)
- tbsp. Lemon juice
- tsp Old Bay seasoning

Directions:

1. Preheat the oven to 400°F. Line a baking sheet using foil or parchment paper.
2. In a pan at medium heat, sauté onion for about 7-10 minutes, until translucent and browned (or cook longer to caramelize if desired).
3. On the other hand, whisk together the mayonnaise, minced garlic, fresh parsley, lemon juice, and Old Bay seasoning.

4. Stir in the sautéed onion. Carefully fold in the lump crab meat, without breaking up the lumps.
5. Place the salmon fillet on the baking sheet. Organize the crab mixture lengthwise down the middle of the salmon. Starting from the thinner sides of the filet, fold over the long way.
6. Mix together the melted butter and lemon zest. Brush the lemon butter at the top of the salmon. Dust lightly with sea salt and black pepper.
7. Bake for at least 16-20 minutes, until the fish flakes easily with a fork. Sprinkle with additional fresh parsley. Cut crosswise into individual filets to serve.

Nutrition: Calories: 243 Fat: 13g Carbs: 1g Protein: 29g

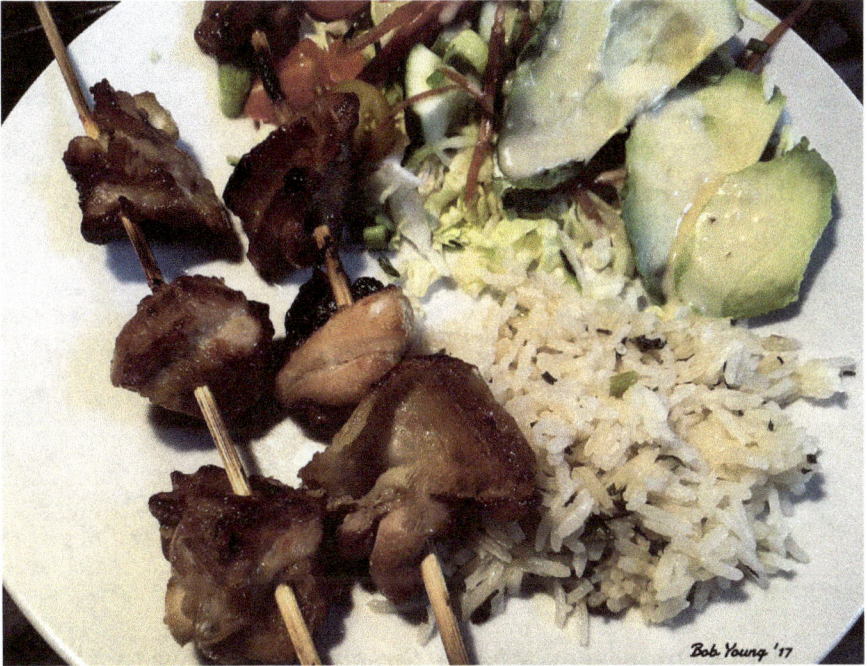

Bob Young '17

Spicy Salmon Tempura Roll

Preparation Time: 10 minutes

Cooking Time: 0 minutes

Servings: 8

Ingredients:

- 4 ounces canned wild salmon
- tbsp. mayonnaise
- 1/2 tbsp. Sirach
- 1/4 tsp ground ginger
- Nori sheet
- 20 grams pork rinds or cracklings
- 1/4 English cucumber, julienned
- 1/2 avocado, sliced into strips
- Sesame seeds (optional)
- Soy sauce (optional)
- Wasabi (optional)
- Pickled ginger (optional)

Directions:

1. Add salmon, mayonnaise, Siracha, and ginger to a bowl and mix until well incorporated.
2. Put pork rinds in a plastic bag and crush until you get large crumbs.
3. Put nori sheet on your work surface with the shiny side down.
4. Combine pork rind crumbs into the salmon mixture.
5. Arrange salmon/pork rind mixture and veggies on the nori, at least an inch away from the edge closest to you.

Roll the nori around the filling tightly, tucking the edge under as you go. Spread a small amount of water on the remaining "rough" side of the nori and continue rolling to bind together and create a uniform roll.

6. Slice in half, then continue to slice every portion in half until you get 8 pieces
7. Garnish with sesame seeds, soy sauce, wasabi or pickled ginger.
8. Serve.

Nutrition: Calories: 243 Fat: 14g Carbs: 6g Protein: 23g

Lemon Butter Tilapia

Preparation Time: 10 minutes

Cooking Time: 10-12 minutes

Servings: 4

Ingredients:

- 1/4 cup unsalted butter, melted
- 3 cloves garlic, minced
- 2 tablespoons freshly squeezed lemon juice
- Zest of 1 lemon
- 4 (6-ounce) tilapia fillets
- Kosher salt, to taste
- Freshly ground black pepper, to taste
- 2 tablespoons chopped fresh parsley leaves

Directions:

1. Set oven to 425°F. Lightly grease using oil a 9×13 baking dish or coat with nonstick spray.
2. In a small bowl, put butter, garlic, lemon juice, and lemon zest, whisk together and set aside.
3. Spice the tilapia with salt and pepper to taste and place onto the prepared baking dish. Drizzle with butter mixture.
4. Bring into the oven and bake until fish flakes easily with a fork, about 10-12 minutes.
5. Serve immediately, garnished with parsley, if desired.

Nutrition: Calories: 276 Fat: 14.5g Carbs: 1.8g Protein: 35.5g

Thai Salmon Fishcakes

Preparation Time: 10 minutes

Cooking Time: 10 minutes

Servings: 2

Ingredients:

- 2 salmon fillets, skin removed
- egg
- tbsp. fresh cilantro roughly chopped
- green onions roughly chopped
- ½ tsp red Thai curry paste
- salt and black pepper to taste

Directions:

1. Set all the ingredients into a food processor and process until smooth.
2. Put some wax paper or baking parchment onto a plate. Divide the mixture into 4, then spoon each portion onto the paper. Cover with another layer of paper and a layer of plastic wrap, and leave in the fridge for at least an hour.
3. Warm, a large non-stick frying pan and fry the fishcakes for 5 minutes at medium heat. Turnover and cook for another five minutes or until cooked through.

Nutrition: Calories: 278 Fat: 12g Carbs: 1g Protein: 36g

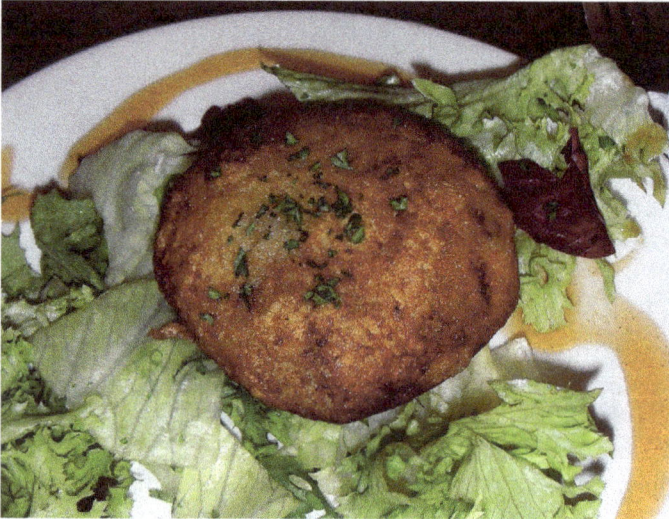

Ahi Tuna Poke

Preparation Time: 10 minutes

Cooking Time: 0 minutes

Servings: 2

Ingredients:

- ½ lbs. Ahi tuna
- Avocado
- scallions
- tbsp. Soy sauce
- tbsp. Sesame oil
- tbsp. Chili garlic sauce
- tbsp. Sesame seeds

Directions:

1. Rinse the ahi tuna and chop it into bite-sized cubes.
2. Rinse the green onions and chop it finely.
3. Combine soy, sesame oil, chili garlic sauce, green onion, and half the sesame seeds in a bowl.
4. Put the ahi to the dressing and mix well. Allow it to sit in the fridge for 10-20 minutes for the flavors to mix.
5. Chop the avocado into small cubes and gently mix it into the rest of the dish right before serving.
6. Sprinkle the remaining sesame seeds on top.
7. Serve with chips or bread and enjoy!

Nutrition: Calories: 350 Fat: 20g Carbs: 9.5g Protein: 30

Vegetables à la Grecque

Preparation time: 2 minutes

Cooking time: 8 minutes

Servings: 4

Ingredients:

- 2 tablespoons olive oil
- 2 garlic cloves, minced
- red onion, chopped
- 10 ounces button mushrooms, thinly sliced
- (1-pound) eggplant, sliced
- 1/2 teaspoon dried basil
- teaspoon dried oregano
- thyme sprig, leaves picked
- rosemary sprigs, leaves picked
- 1/2 cup tomato sauce
- 1/4 cup dry Greek wine
- 1/4 cup water
- 8 ounces Halloumi cheese, cubed
- tablespoons Kalamata olives, pitted and halved

Directions:

1. Press the "Sauté" button to heat up your Instant Pot; now, heat the olive oil. Cook the garlic and red onions for 1 to 2 minutes, stirring periodically.

2. Stir in the mushrooms and continue to sauté an additional 2 to 3 minutes.
3. Add the eggplant, basil, oregano, thyme, rosemary, tomato sauce, Greek wine, and water.
4. Secure the lid. Choose "Manual" mode and Low pressure; cook for 3 minutes. Once cooking is complete, use a quick pressure release; carefully remove the lid.
5. Top with cheese and olives. Bon appétit!

Nutrition: 326 Calories; 25.1g Fat; 8.4g Carbs; 15.7g Protein; 4.3g Sugars

Spinach artichoke egg casserole

Preparation time: 10 minutes

Cooking time: 35 minutes

Servings: 12

Ingredients:

- Milk (¼ cup)
- Shredded white cheddar (1 cup)
- Eggs (16)
- Frozen chopped spinach (10 ounces)
- Ricotta cheese (½ cup)
- Drained artichoke hearts (1 can)
- Parmesan cheese (½ cup)
- Shaved onions (¼ cup)
- Dried thyme (½ tsp)
- Minced garlic (1 clove)
- Salt (1 tsp)
- Crushed red pepper (½ tsp)

Directions:

1. Prep your oven by heating to 350°F.
2. Prep a baking dish by coating it with nonstick cooking spray.
3. Crack the eggs into a bowl and whisk with milk.
4. Break or cut the artichoke hearts into tiny bits and remove the leaves.
5. Remove all the excess water from the spinach and add it to the eggs and milk along with the tiny artichokes.

6. Now add all the other ingredients except the ricotta cheese. Stir to mix.
7. Gently pour this mixture into the baking dish.
8. Dollop ricotta cheese over the egg casserole. Make this as even as possible.
9. Slide the dish into the oven and leave for about 35 minutes. When the pan stops jiggling when you shake it, it's ready.
10. Serve

Nutrition: 230 calories. Fats: 16g Carbs: 4g Protein:16g Fiber : 1g

Broccoli and Cheese Fritters

Preparation time: 2 minutes

Cooking time: 8 minutes

Servings: 16

Ingredients:

- Fritters:
- Fresh broccoli (4 ounces)
- Almond flour (¾ cup)
- Mozzarella chèese (4 ounces)
- Flaxseed meal (¼ cup)
- Eggs (2)
- Salt
- Baking soda (2 tsp)
- Pepper
- Sauce:
- Chopped dill(¼ cup)
- Salt
- Lemon juice (½ tbsp)
- Mayonnaise (¼ cup)
- Pepper

Directions:

1. Take the broccoli through a food processor. When it's completely broken down, set aside.
2. Mix the mozzarella, a quarter of flaxseed meal, almond flour and bacon powder together and pour it into the bowl with the broccoli. This is the time to add all the

seasoning you want so if there's anything you'd like to add, do it here.

3. Break and beat the eggs. Pour it into the broccoli mix and stir.
4. Make little balls out of the mix and roll it in the remaining flaxseed meal to coat.
5. Preheat your deep fat fryer to 375°F.
6. When it's hot, put your fritters inside and fry until it looks golden. This should take 5 minutes.
7. Put the fritters in a bed of paper towels to drain the excess oil.
8. Prepare your sauce with zesty dill, lemon and mayonnaise.
9. Serve.

Nutrition: 78 calories Fat: 5.8g Carbs: 1.3g Protein: 4.6g

With sauce: 1 serving contains 103.9 calories. Fat: 8.35g Carbs: 1.89g Protein: 4.57g

Garlic and Chive Cauliflower Mash

Preparation time: 5 minutes

Cooking time: 15 minutes

Servings: 1

Ingredients:

- Peeled garlic (1 clove)
- Cauliflower florets (4 cups)
- Water (1 tablespoon)
- Mayonnaise (⅓ cup)
- Kosher salt (½ teaspoon)
- Lemon juice (¼ teaspoon)
- Chopped chives (1 tablespoon)
- Black pepper (⅛ teaspoon)
- Lime zest (½ teaspoon)

Directions:

1. Get a large bowl and throw in all the ingredients except the lime zest, lemon juice and chives. Mix thoroughly.
2. Put this in a microwave for 15 minutes or longer. Depends on how soft you want it to be.
3. Put this cooked mix through a food processor until it is smooth.
4. Throw in the chives, lemon juice and lime zest and put it through the food processor again.
5. Serve warm.

Nutrition: ½ serving contains 178 calories. Fat: 18g Carbs: 3g Protein: 2g

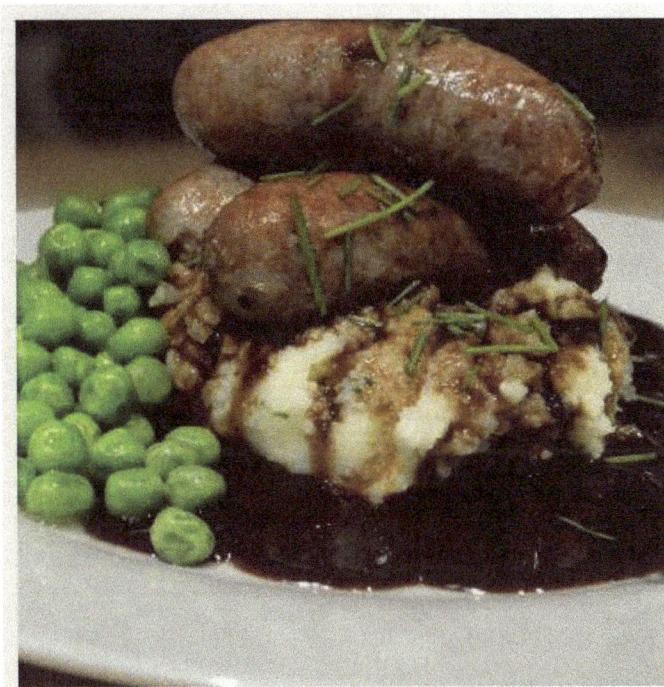

SOUPS AND STEWS

Slow Cooker Beer Soup with Cheddar & Sausage

Preparation Time: 20 minutes

Cooking Time: 8 hours

Servings: 8

Ingredients:

- cup heavy cream
- 10 ounces sausages, sliced
- cup celery, chopped
- cup carrots, chopped
- 4 garlic cloves, minced
- 8 ounces cream cheese
- tsp red pepper flakes
- 6 ounces beer
- 16 ounces beef stock
- onion, diced
- cup cheddar cheese, grated
- Salt and black pepper, to taste
- Fresh cilantro, chopped, to garnish

Directions:

1. Turn on the slow cooker. Add beef stock, beer, sausages, carrots, onion, garlic, celery, salt, red pepper flakes, and black pepper, and stir to combine. Pour in enough water

to cover all the ingredients by roughly 2 inches. Close the lid and cook for 6 hours on Low.

2. Open the lid and stir in the heavy cream, cheddar, and cream cheese, and cook for 2 more hours. Ladle the soup into bowls and garnish with cilantro before serving. Yummy!

Nutrition: Calories: 244 Fat,: 17g Net Carbs: 4g Protein: 5g

Beef Reuben Soup

Preparation Time: 10 minutes

Cooking Time: 20 minutes

Servings: 6

Ingredients:

- onion, diced
- 6 cups beef stock
- tsp caraway seeds
- celery stalks, diced
- garlic cloves, minced
- cups heavy cream
- cup sauerkraut, shredded
- pound corned beef, chopped
- tbsp. butter
- ½ cup swiss cheese, shredded
- Salt and black pepper, to taste

Directions:

1. Melt the butter in a large pot. Add onion and celery, and fry for 3 minutes until tender. Add garlic and cook for another minute.
2. Pour the beef stock over and stir in sauerkraut, salt, caraway seeds, and add a pinch of black pepper. Bring to a boil. Reduce the heat to low, and add the corned beef. Cook for about 15 minutes, adjust the seasoning. Stir in heavy cream and cheese and cook for 1 minute.

Nutrition: Calories: 450 Fat,: 37g Net Carbs: 8g Protein: 23g

Coconut, Green Beans & Shrimp Curry Soup

Preparation Time: 10 minutes

Cooking Time: 15 minutes

Servings: 4

Ingredients:

- 2 tbsp. ghee
- lb. jumbo shrimp, peeled and deveined
- tsp ginger-garlic puree
- tbsp. red curry paste
- 6 oz. coconut milk
- Salt and chili pepper to taste
- bunch green beans, halved

Directions:

1. Melt ghee in a medium saucepan over medium heat. Add the shrimp, season with salt and black pepper, and cook until they are opaque, 2 to 3 minutes. Remove shrimp to a plate. Add the ginger-garlic puree and red curry paste to the ghee and sauté for 2 minutes until fragrant.
2. Stir in the coconut milk; add the shrimp, salt, chili pepper, and green beans. Cook for 4 minutes. Reduce the heat to a simmer and cook an additional 3 minutes, occasionally stirring. Adjust taste with salt, fetch soup into serving bowls, and serve with cauli rice.

Nutrition: Calories 375 Fat 35.4g Net Carbs 2g Protein 9g

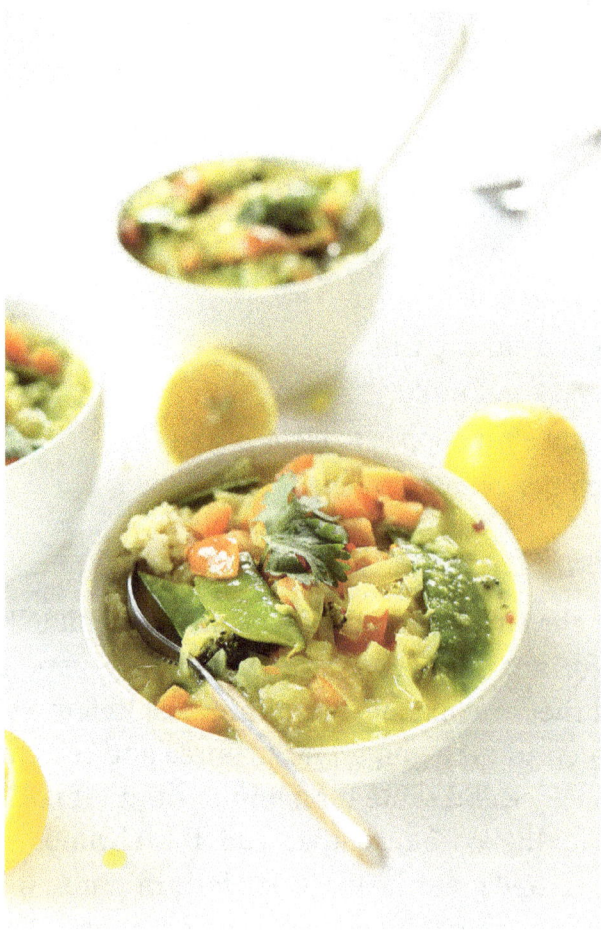

Brazilian Moqueca (Shrimp Stew)

Preparation Time: 10 minutes

Cooking Time: 15 minutes

Servings: 6

Ingredients:

- cup coconut milk
- tbsp. lime juice
- ¼ cup diced roasted peppers
- ½ pounds shrimp, peeled and deveined
- ¼ cup olive oil
- garlic clove, minced
- 14 ounces diced tomatoes
- tbsp. sriracha sauce
- chopped onion
- ¼ cup chopped cilantro
- Fresh dill, chopped to garnish
- Salt and black pepper, to taste

Directions:

1. Heat the olive oil in a pot over medium heat. Add onion and cook for 3 minutes or until translucent. Add the garlic and cook for another minute, until soft. Add tomatoes, shrimp, and cilantro. Cook until the shrimp becomes opaque, about 3-4 minutes.
2. Stir in sriracha sauce and coconut milk, and cook for 2 minutes. Do not bring to a boil. Stir in the lime juice and season with salt and pepper. Spoon the stew in bowls, garnish with fresh dill to serve.

Nutrition: Calories: 324 Fat: 21g, Net Carbs: 5g Protein: 23.1g

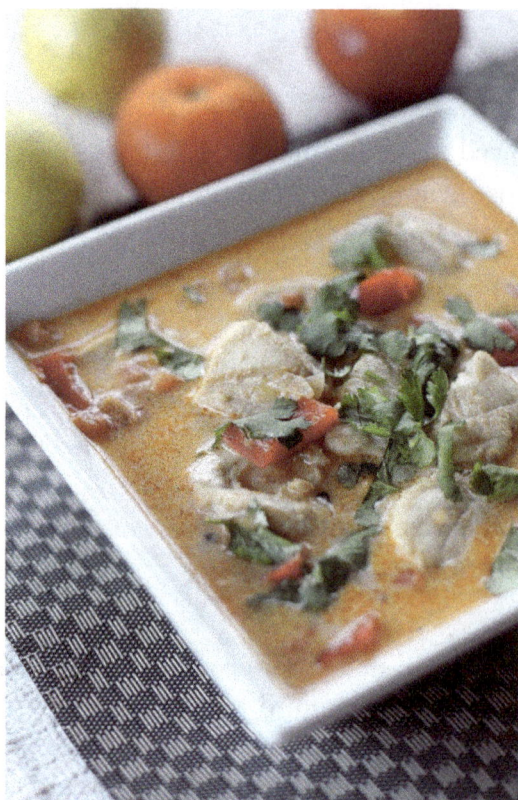

SNACKS

Spicy Bacon and Avocado Balls

Preparation time: 45 minutes

Cooking time: 8 minutes

Servings: 6

Ingredients:

- 4 slices bacon
- medium avocado
- Tbsp coconut oil
- Tbsp bacon fat
- Tbsp green onions, finely chopped
- Tbsp cilantro, finely chopped
- small jalapeño pepper, seeded, finely chopped
- ¼ tsp sea salt

Directions:

1. Over medium heat, cook bacon until golden, about 4 minutes each side.
2. Drain bacon on a paper towel. Save bacon fat for later.
3. Once bacon is cool, chop 2 slices into crumbles.
4. Cut remaining 2 slices into 3 pieces each.
5. Smash avocado with a fork in a small bowl.
6. Add coconut oil and cooled bacon fat to avocado.
7. Add onion, cilantro, jalapeño, salt, and bacon crumbles. Blend well.

8. Refrigerate for 30 minutes.
9. Form mixture into 6 balls.
10. Place remaining 6 bacon pieces on a plate, then top each with an avocado ball.
11. Serve or refrigerate up to 3 days.

Nutrition: Total Carbs – 3 g Net Carbs – 1 g Fat – 18 g Protein – 3 g Calories – 181

Brie Cheese Fat Bombs

Preparation time: 15 minutes

Cooking time: 3 minutes

Servings: 6

Ingredients:

- 2 oz full-fat cream cheese
- ¼ cup unsalted butter
- ½ cup Brie cheese, chopped
- tbsp ghee
- white onion, diced
- garlic clove, minced
- ½ tsp paprika
- Salt, pepper to taste
- 6 lettuce leaves

Directions:

1. In a food processor, mix the cream cheese and butter. Transfer to a bowl. Mix in the Brie.
2. In a pan, add onion and garlic and cook 3 minutes over medium heat with ghee. Let cool. Once cooled, combine with the cheese and butter mixture.
3. Season with the spices and mix. Refrigerate 30 minutes.
4. Make 6 fat bombs out of the mixture. Serve on lettuce leaves.

Nutrition: Total Carbs – 1.7 g Net Carbs –1.4 g Fat – 16.2 g Protein – 3.3 g Calories – 158

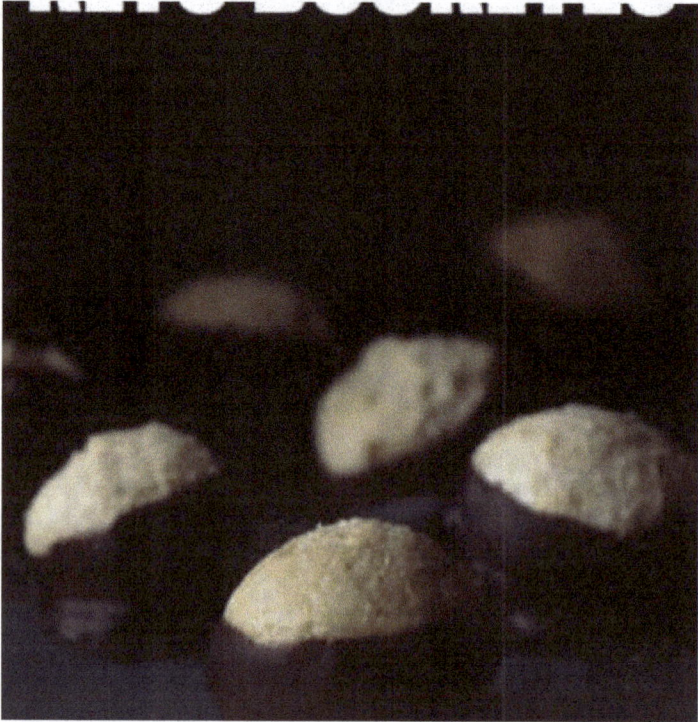

Salted Caramel and Brie Balls

Preparation time: 5 minutes

Cooking time: 5 minutes

Servings: 6

Ingredients:

- 4 oz Brie, roughly chopped
- 2 oz salted macadamia nuts
- ½ tsp caramel flavor
- Tbsp butter
- large apple, chopped

Directions:

1. In a food processor, mix all ingredients until a coarse mix forms, about 30 seconds.
2. Form mixture into 6 balls.
3. In a saucepan, melt the butter, then add the chopped apples. Cook until apples for about 5 minutes.
4. Spoon the apples over the brie balls. Serve or refrigerate up to 3 days.

Nutrition: Total Carbs – 1 g Net Carbs – 0 g Fat – 12 g Protein – 5 g Calories – 130

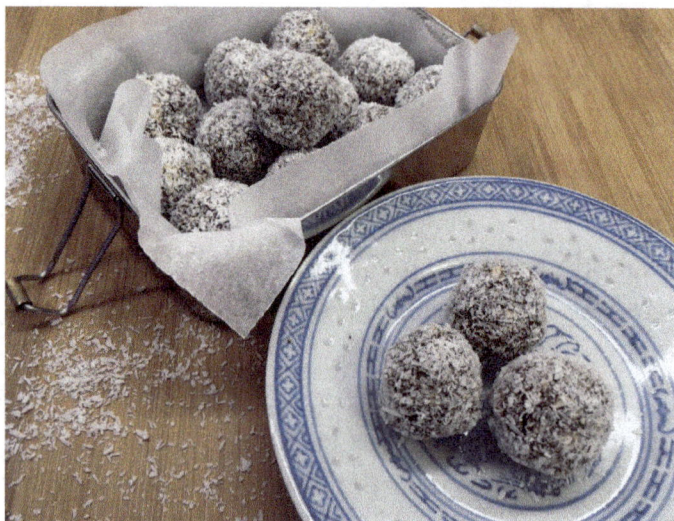

SMOOTHIES AND DRINKS

Cinnamon Raspberry Smoothie

Preparation Time: 11 minutes

Cooking Time: 0 minutes

Servings: 1

Ingredients:

- cup of unsweetened almond milk
- 1/2 cup of frozen raspberries
- cup of spinach or kale
- tbsp. of almond butter
- 1/8 tsp of cinnamon, or more to taste

Directions:

1. Place all the ingredients into the blender and blend until pureed.
2. Enjoy as breakfast or snacks.

Nutrition: 286 calories 21g fat 19g carbohydrates 10g protein

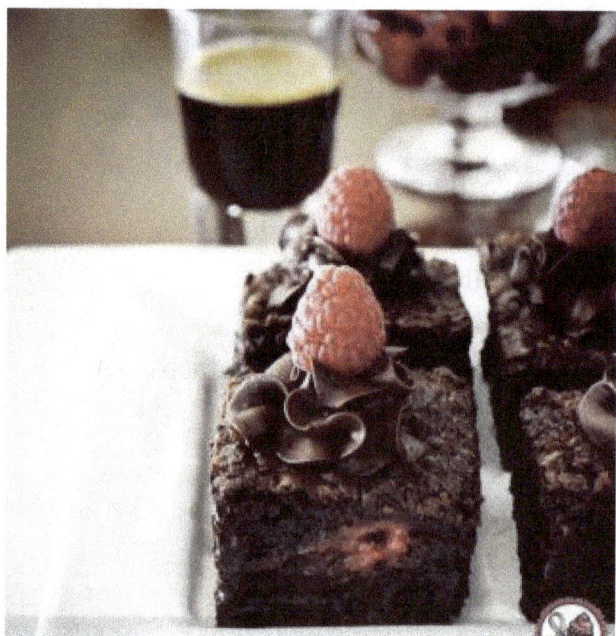

DESSERTS

Butter Pecan Ice Cream

Preparation time: 5 minutes

Cooking time: 5 minutes

Servings: 3

Ingredients:

- ½ cups unsweetened coconut milk
- ¼ cup heavy whipping cream
- 5 tbsp butter
- ¼ cup crushed pecans
- 25 drops liquid stevia
- ¼ tsp xanthan gum

Directions:

1. Place a pan over medium-low heat and melt butter in it until it turns brown.
2. Mix this butter with chopped pecans, heavy cream, and stevia in a bowl.
3. Stir in coconut milk then xanthan gum and mix well until fluffy.
4. Add this mixture to an ice cream machine and churn as per the machine's instructions.
5. Once done, serve.

Nutrition: Calories 251 Total Fat 24.5 g Saturated Fat 14.7 g Cholesterol 165 mg Sodium 142 mg Total Carbs 4.3 g Sugar 0.5 g   Fiber 1 g Protein 5.9 g

Almond Meal Cupcakes

Preparation time: 15 minutes

Cooking time: 15 minutes

Servings: 12

Ingredients:

- ½ cup almond meal
- ¼ cup butter, melted
- 2 (8-ounce / 227-g) packages cream cheese, softened
- 2 eggs
- ¾ teaspoon liquid stevia
- teaspoon vanilla extract
- Special equipment:
- A 12-cup muffin pan

Directions:

1. Preheat your oven to 350°F (180°C). Line a muffin pan with 12 paper liners.
2. Thoroughly mix the almond meal with butter in a bowl, then spoon this mixture into the bottoms of each paper liner and press it into a thin crust.
3. Make the cupcakes: Whisk the cream cheese with liquid stevia, eggs, and vanilla extract in a medium bowl. Beat with an electric beater until the mixture is fluffy, creamy and smooth. Spoon this filling over the crust layer in the muffin pan.
4. Bake in the preheated oven until the cream cheese mixture is cooked from the center, for 15 to 17 minutes.

5. Leave the cupcakes to cool at room temperature. Serve immediately or refrigerate to chill for 8 hours, preferably overnight.

Nutrition: calories: 199 fat: 19.1g total carbs: 2.6g fiber: 0.5g protein: 4.7g

Almond Cinnamon Cookies

Preparation time: 10 minutes

Cooking time: 15 minutes

Servings: 12

Ingredients:

- 2 cups blanched almond flour
- ½ cup butter, softened
- egg
- ½ cup Swerve
- teaspoon sugar-free vanilla extract
- teaspoon ground cinnamon

Directions:

1. Preheat your oven to 350°F (180°C). Layer a baking sheet with parchment paper.
2. Whisk the almond flour with butter, vanilla extract, Swerve, egg, and cinnamon in a bowl. Mix well until these ingredients form a smooth dough.
3. Make the cookies: Divide the dough and roll it into 1-inch balls on a lightly floured surface. Arrange these balls on the prepared baking sheet and press each ball lightly with a fork to make a crisscross pattern.
4. Bake these cinnamon cookies in the preheated oven for 12 to 15 minutes, or until their edges turn golden.
5. Allow the cinnamon cookies to cool on the baking sheet for 5 minutes, then transfer them to a wire rack to cool completely before serving.

Nutrition: calories: 92 fat: 7.4g total carbs: 3.0g fiber: 0.1g protein: 3.4g

CPSIA information can be obtained
at www.ICGtesting.com
Printed in the USA
BVHW092054190421
605311BV00002B/39

9 781802 331509